Intermittent Fasting
for Women:

Burn Fat in Less Than 30 Days with Serious Permanent Weight Loss in Very Simple, Healthy and Easy Scientific Way, Eat More Food and Lose More Weight

Table of Contents

Furthermore, the transmission, duplication or reproduction of any of the following work including specific information will be considered an illegal act irrespective of if it is done electronically or in print. This extends to creating a secondary or tertiary copy of the work or a recorded copy and is only allowed with express written consent from the Publisher. All additional right reserved.

The information in the following pages is broadly considered to be a truthful and accurate account of facts and as such any inattention, use or misuse of the information in question by the reader will render any resulting actions solely under their purview. There are no scenarios in which the publisher or the original author of this work can be in any fashion deemed liable for any hardship or damages that may befall them after undertaking information described herein.

Additionally, the information in the following pages is intended only for informational purposes and should thus be thought of as universal. As befitting its nature, it is presented without assurance regarding its prolonged validity or interim quality. Trademarks that are mentioned are done without written consent and can in no way be considered an endorsement from the trademark holder.

Introduction

Congratulations on downloading *Intermittent Fasting for Women: Burn Fat in Less Than 30 Days with Serious Permanent Weight Loss in Very Simple, Healthy and Easy Scientific Way, Eat More Food and Lose More Weight* and thank you for doing so. Intermittent fasting has been practiced around the world for thousands of years so regardless of why you have decided to try this diet, rest assured that you are in good company.

Just because the path is well trod doesn't make it easy to follow, however, especially if you find you aren't always in control as far as food is concerned which is why this book will provide you with everything you need to get started in the most effective way possible. First, you will learn the basics of intermittent fasting, the history of the process and how to get started successfully. Next, you will learn about the unique concerns that women have to watch out for when practicing intermittent fasting as well as what you can do to mitigate them as thoroughly as possible.

From there, you will learn all about several types of intermittent fasting including the 4:3 or 5:2 method, the eat-stop-eat method, the Leangains method, the forever fat loss method and the alternate fasting method. You will find pros and cons associated with each as well as how to give each a fair shake in order to see what types of fasting work best for you. You will then learn about how to add exercise to your intermittent fasting plan and how to ensure you don't have to sacrifice tone and definition just because you are fasting. Finally, you will find a variety of tips to ensure you blast through the transition phase and create new long-term habits as easily as possible.

The following chapters will discuss

There are plenty of books on this subject on the market, thanks again for choosing this one! Every effort was made to ensure it is full of as much useful information as possible, please enjoy!

Chapter 1: Fasting Basics

The practice of intermittent fasting has been around for countless centuries and used for nearly as many different purposes. However, the reason that most people have heard about the practice these days is thanks to its proven ability to help those who practice it lose weight and keep it off in the long-term while at the same time feeling more energized than they have in years.

The best part? Getting into the intermittent fasting lifestyle doesn't require you to give up the foods you love or even eat fewer calories per meal. In fact, the most commonly used type of intermittent fasting makes it possible for those who practice it to skip breakfast before eating two meals later in the day. This type of lifestyle change is ideal for those who find themselves having trouble sticking with a stricter diet plan as it doesn't take much of a change to start seeing serious results, as opposed to being forced to change everything all at once. In fact, this is what makes intermittent fasting a great choice for both the long and short-term as it is easy enough to get started with and stick with in the long-term and also effective enough to generate continual results so that those who practice it are motivated to keep up their good work.

The reason that intermittent fasting is so successful is because of the incontrovertible truth that your body behaves differently when it is in a fed state as opposed to when it is in a fasting state. A fed state is any period of time when your body is currently absorbing nutrients from food while digesting it. This state starts about five minutes after you have finished your meal and will stick around for as many as five hours depending on the type of meal it was and how difficult it is for your body to break it down into energy. While your body is in this state it is constantly producing insulin, which makes it far more difficult for the body to burn fat than it is when insulin production is not taking place.

The next state occurs directly following digestion before the fasted state has occurred. It is known as the buffer period and it will then last anywhere between eight and 12 hours based on what you last ate and personal body chemistry. It is only during this state, once your insulin levels have returned to normal that your body will be able to burn fat at peak efficiency. Due to the amount of time required to reach a true fasting state, many people never feel its full effects as they rarely go eight hours without eating, much less 12. This doesn't mean making the transition is impossible, however, all you need to do is ensure you take advantage of this natural state as a way of breaking the three squares a day habit.

A historical practice

As a tradition, intermittent fasting is even older than the written word. While using it primarily as a means of weight loss can be considered a relatively new phenomenon, it has a long history of use for things like divine communication, disease prevention, improving concentration, reducing the signs of aging and more. Fasting has been used by practically every religion and culture since the invention of agriculture.

Hippocrates, perhaps the founding father of modern medicine was practicing his trade around 400 BC and one of the most commonly prescribed treatments was of fasting regularly and drinking apple cider vinegar. He believed (rightly so) that eating takes away essential resources via the digestive process that the body could otherwise use for more productive processes as well. This idea came about because Hippocrates study the natural inclination of all mammals to ignore food while they are sick.

Paracelsus, a contemporary of Hippocrates and the creator of the study of toxicology felt the same way, going so far as to refer to the process of fasting as the "physician within" because of all the potential for good it can do in the human body. This tenant was then later expanded upon even more by none other than Benjamin Franklin who believed that intermittent fasting was one of the best ways to cure a host of common ailments.

Religious practices: Fasting of one sort or another has always been seen by some as a spiritual practice which is likely why it is a major tenant for religions around the world. Everyone from Buddha, to Muhammed, to Jesus Christ were all known to preach the benefits of fasting on a regular schedule. The idea here is that the aim of the practice is to purify the physical or spiritual self, likely due to the increase in mental clarity the process provides, with a dash of its healing power thrown in for good measure. In fact, many

Buddhists regularly eat in the morning and then fast to the morning of the next day in order to feel even closer to their faith. Water fasts that get longer and longer as the practitioner ages are also quite common.

When it comes to Christianity, numerous different sects fast for strict lengths of time for similar reasons. The most extreme example of this is perhaps the Greek Orthodox Christians who fast for as many as 200 days out of the year. It is important to note that the Mediterranean Diet, which made it well known how healthy people are in that region, based much of it research in Crete which is largely Greek Orthodox. As such, it is highly likely that intermittent fasting should be a natural part of this diet as well.

In the largest branch of Christianity, Roman Catholicism, fasting is traditional observed at several key points through the year and is generally practiced by eating one large meal in the middle of the day as well as two smaller meals at a time that is close to the first meal. This is most commonly observed on Ash Wednesday, which includes not eating any meat, and all the Fridays in the month of Lent. While this is not required, it is requested by those who are older than 18 and under 59. This practice as followed today is far less strict than it once was prior to 1956.

Besides these days, Roman Catholics are expected to follow the event known by the name the Eucharistic Fast. This is the fast that is supposed to take place 60 minutes prior to the time the practitioner knows they will be taking mass. This timeframe used to extend between 12 am and the time of Mass on Saturday but was shortened to the point where it doesn't provide any real benefits except to get the body used to not eating.

In the Bahai faith, practitioners practice fasting each day for 12 hours during the month of March and they abstain from liquids in addition to foods.

Everyone in the faith between the ages of 15 and 70 is expected to participate if they feel they can do it properly. Fasting is also regularly seen as part of the Muslim faith during Ramadan. This is a similar daylight fast that even excludes water. The prophet Muhammad was also known to encourage regular intermittent fasting as well.

Fasting is also an important part of the Hindu religion as it asks its followers to observe several different types of fasts based on local custom and person belief. It is common for many Hindus to fast certain days of each month including Purnima, Pradosha or Ekadasi. Additionally, the individual days of the week are also dedicated to fasting based on which deity the practitioner is devoted to. Those who worship Shiva typically fast on Mondays, followers of Vishnu tend to fast on Thursdays and followers of Ayyappa typically fast on Saturdays.

Fasting is also a common part of life in India where they regularly fast on specific days. In many parts of the country, they fast on Tuesdays in respect of the goddess Mariamman, one of the forms of the goddess Shakti or Lord Hanuman. This is a liquid only fast for the day though some followers will consume fruit as well.

Intermittent fasting benefits

The fasting state is ideal when it comes to losing weight and building muscle, but these are only two of the primary benefits of intermittent fasting. One of the most unexpected benefits for many people is the amount of time you will end up saving when you suddenly don't have to worry about eating an entire meal, especially if you take the traditional route and cut out breakfast, freeing up crucial time in what is often the most hectic part of the day for many people. Along similar lines, you will also find that you have extra money in your food budget as breakfast foods are often some of the priciest as well. The difference will likely be noticeable, even if you eat a little bit more throughout the rest of the day as well.

While the idea of giving up an entire meal every day might seem unthinkable now, with practice you will be surprised at how manageable it will become. It will certainly be worth it as well because, in addition to ensuring there is extra time in your day and extra money in your bank account, it can quite literally help you live a longer, healthier life. In fact, studies show that when you spend extra time in the fasted state your body diverts that energy to its core survival systems in much the same way it would when you are starving. While your body might view them as the same in the short-term, the fact of the matter is that the two states are extremely different which means that the end result is that your body ends up rejuvenated by the process as opposed to being sustained.

Specifically, if you spend a prolonged period of time in a fasted state you will greatly reduce your risk of stroke along with your risk of a wide variety of cardiovascular issues. It has also been proven to lessen the effects of chemotherapy in cancer patients as well. What's more, these health benefits don't take months or years to appear, they start to emerge as soon as you get into the habit of intermittent fasting and decrease your overall caloric intake by more than 15 percent. Even more, benefits materialize in the form of improvements to reproductive organ and kidney function, blood pressure, oxidative resistance and glucose tolerance.

While all the nitty gritty as to why skipping a few meals, each day leads to such dramatic benefits isn't clear, what scientists have determined is that it is related to the reduction of repetitive stress that the body experiences while fasting as opposed to eating three large meals a day. This is also why it improves the health of the digestive tract as well as that of many important organs. It even gives the mitochondria in your body a boost, ensuring they utilize the energy available to them as efficiently as possible. This, in turn, has the added beneficial effect of decreasing the odds of oxidation damage occurring anywhere in the system.

The health benefits to the body are notable enough that both alternate days fasting, and many forms of intermittent fasting are a medically approved way of decreasing one's risk of developing type 2 diabetes for those who are already experiencing the symptoms of pre-diabetes. Now, this benefit can certainly be negated, which is why it is important to not use the fact that you are fasting as an excuse to eat everything and anything that you want, some self-control will still be required. This is why the best choice is to not treat your time fasting as some great feat, but to instead act as though it is just a regular part of your routine.

To understand just how effective intermittent fasting can be, consider an experiment that was performed on yeast cells that found when the yeast was deprived of food its cells began to divide more slowly in response. When applied to your cells what this means is that while you are fasting each of your cells literally lives longer than would otherwise be the case thanks to this artificial scarcity.

While the above list of health benefits should be enough to at least make most people think twice about intermittent fasting before dismissing it outright, once they get started many people are surprised to find that one of the things they enjoy most about the intermittent fasting process is the fact that it is such a simple yet productive addition to their day. It is so easy to use, in fact, that in a study of those more than 30 pounds overweight, it was found that more participants were able to stick to an intermittent fasting plan than any other over a three-month period of time.

What's more, while they were practicing intermittent fasting, this group of individuals saw the same overall amount of weight loss as anyone else. Perhaps most encouraging of all, however, is that a year after the study had been completed, more of those who had been intermittent fasting were still with it compared to the others and they had unilaterally lost the most weight overall.

Getting started

With so many benefits out there, you may be understandably anxious to get started for yourself. In order to ensure you are able to stick with the practice of intermittent fasting for the long-term, however, there are a few guidelines you should keep in mind.

Burn more than you eat: While the idea that you need to burn more calories than you consume is far from revolutionary, it is especially important to keep it in mind while you are fasting intermittently as it can be far easier to overeat post-fast than would otherwise be the case, especially when you are still getting used to the process. If you do slip, it can be easy to undue all of your hard work for the day with just a few misplaced bites.

There are 3,500 calories in a pound which means that each week you need to burn a minimum of 3,500 calories compared to what you consume if you want to keep up your weight loss on a regular basis. While you may experience a period where you are losing more than that as your body adjusts to the new style of eating, a steady one pound a week is the ideal amount as anything more than that is unstainable in the long-term without eventually putting your health at risk.

Always remain in control: In order to use intermittent fasting effectively, it is vital that you have an appropriate relationship with food right from the start. If you are the type of person who feels as though certain foods, especially their favorite foods have a pull over them and your willpower goes out the window at the site of them then you may have a hard time getting started with intermittent fasting. Remember, it is vital that you have the willpower to go a minimum of 12 hours without eating as any caloric intake is going to be enough to start generating insulin and thus reset the clock. You need to be able to cut out 500 calories from your diet, per day, in order to lose a pound a week.

Recommendation: Download the app "myfitnesspal" to your smartphone it will help you *estimate* how many calories you should consume every day, you can add and log recipes from across the web.

While ensuring that you don't eat too much is a vital part of the process, it is only half the battle as the other half is ensuring that you don't let yourself go too long without eating. If you intend to make intermittent fasting part of your life in the long-term then it is vital that you learn how to add it to your life in a healthy fashion as going to far in one direction or the other is only going to lead to failure and potentially serious health problems.

Stick with it: When it comes to using intermittent fasting regularly, it is important to find the variation that works best for you and then settle into a long-term routine as opposed to starting and stopping regularly. While you are sure to see some results right away, it will take about a month for your body to fully adjust to the process which means you need to be committed to the cause and patient as well as nothing happens overnight. While you are sure to find yourself extremely hungry, at first, after your body has learned when it can start expecting calories you will find that your hunger more or less returns to normal. Furthermore, a month should be enough time to start seeing physical results as well which should be enough to buffer your mental fortitude even more.

On the other hand, if you rapidly switch between methods of intermittent fasting, or only use it for short bursts now and then, then rather than enhance your body's ability to lose weight naturally while also building muscle, you will instead find it difficult to much of anything effectively as your body will be in a constant state of confusion. As such, all weight loss will cease as it tries to hang on to every single calorie possible until it can figure out what in the world is going on. If you truly hope to see the types of results you are looking then the best way to ensure this is the case is to find one schedule of eating that works for you and then stick with it.

Talk to a healthcare professional: While its true that intermittent fasting helps people to lose weight and build muscle, in addition to a host of other benefits, this doesn't mean it is automatically for everyone or that it doesn't come along with some side effects as well. For starters, when you first transition to an intermittent fasting lifestyle you are likely to experience diarrhea, constipation or episodes of both for the first two weeks or so as your body adjusts to its new habits.

Furthermore, it is important to be very careful in not letting yourself binge after you have finished fasting as this can lead to internal damage as well. Regardless of how healthy you plan to be; however, it is important that you talk your plans over with either a dietitian or healthcare professional to ensure you don't end up accidentally doing yourself more harm than good.

Chapter 2: Women and Intermittent Fasting

While intermittent fasting is beneficial for both men and women, men's bodies do take to the transition more easily than women's bodies do. As such, as a woman, if you hope to make intermittent fasting a healthy part of your lifestyle then there are a few additional things you need to keep in mind.

Many women who have tried intermittent fasting acknowledge its numerous benefits. These include reduced risks of heart disease, gaining lean muscle, recommended blood sugar levels, reduced risk of chronic diseases such as cancer and many others. However, along with the good come hormonal changes within their bodies that bring with them some other changes to an active lifestyle.

Nutrition deficiency: When adopting an intermittent fasting lifestyle, the first thing women need to keep in mind is that the transition phase is likely going to interrupt the body's natural fertility cycle. This is a defensive mechanism that is only discarded when an adequate level of nutrition intake resumes. While fasting can affect your hormones, intermittent fasting does support proper hormonal balance leading to a healthy body and weight loss the right way once the body adjusts to the new way of eating.

Additional challenges: While it is not something that is going to affect everyone, some women who regularly practice intermittent fasting do see problems such as metabolic disturbances, early-onset menopause, and missed periods. In addition, if you find your body experiencing prolonged hormonal issues it could ultimately lead to pale skin, hair loss, acne, decreased energy and the other, similar issues. As long as you don't take your fasting to the extreme, then after the first month or so you should not expect to see any of these issues.

The reason these hormonal imbalances occur is that women are extremely sensitive to what are known as starvation signals. As such, when a woman's body senses that it is not receiving enough vital nutrients it produces an extreme amount of the hormone's leptin and ghrelin in order to increase the woman's desire to eat. As such, if you find that you are absolutely ravenous when you reach the end of your fasting phase then this very well could be the reason why.

The reason that women are so much more susceptible to this issue than men is largely based on a protein called kisspeptin which is used by neurons to aid in communication. It is also extremely sensitive to ghrelin, leptin and insulin and present in far greater quantities in women than in men.

When the body produces excessive hormones that prompt you to eat, you are likely to ignore them. Apparently, many women ignore these hunger signals, so the signals get even more intense. The problem is that even these loud signals are ignored, and this might lead to bingeing which can lead to the creation of a cycle that does little to ensure your body receives the vital nutrients it needs while hurting it in more ways than one. If the negative habits persist for too long, it is possible that it can throw your hormones out of whack permanently.

Metabolism concerns: Your metabolism is intimately tied to your health which means that if you are experiencing physiological or physical challenges, then your health could also be at risk. Luckily, maintaining a healthy diet while exercising, working out and fasting regularly can all help to resolve these types of health challenges. Over time, intermittent fasting has even shown to help balance out hormones which means you just need to be aware of the issue and ride it out while your body adjusts to your new habits.

Protein concerns: Women tend to consume less protein compared to men. It follows then that fasting women consume even less protein. Less consumption of protein results in fewer amino acids in the body. Amino acids are essential for the synthesis of insulin-like growth factor in the liver which activates estrogen receptors. The growth factor IGF-1 causes the uterine wall lining to thicken as well as the progression of the reproductive cycle.

A prolonged low protein intake can also affect your estrogen levels, which can also affect your metabolic function and vice versa. This can potentially affect your mood, digestion, cognition, bone formation and more. It can even affect the brain as estrogen is required to stimulate the neurons responsible for ceasing the production of the chemicals that regulate appetite. Essentially, any time your estrogen levels drop noticeably you are likely to end up feeling hungrier than would otherwise be the case.

Ideal starter intermittent fasting guide for women

As previously discussed, women are naturally more sensitive to feelings of hunger than men are which is why many women find that fasting can be such a challenge. Luckily, there is a variation of intermittent fasting that has been designed to onboard women more easily into an intermittent fasting lifestyle. It is known as Crescendo Fasting and to follow it, all you need to do is start by fasting three days a week on nonconsecutive days.

You will find that you still see many of the overall benefits of intermittent fasting, without subjecting yourself to the potential for hormonal imbalance. This approach is far more gentle on the body during the transition period and it can help you adjust to fasting as quickly as possible. If you still find that you are having issues, then you can start your day with around 250 calories before proceeding to continue your fast as normal.

Benefits: The benefits of this style of intermittent fasting are mostly in line with what the more rigorous versions boast and include:

- You gain energy

- Improving inflammatory markers

- Losing weight and body fat

- No hormonal challenges

Crescendo Fasting Rules: First and foremost, it is important that you don't fast more than three days a week for the first month and never fast for more than 24 hours at a time. During these fasting periods you are going to want to fast anywhere between 12 and 16 hours, it is very important that you never exceed more than 16 hours of fasting at a time if you can help it. On the days that you do fast, you are still going to want to exercise, just do something light or wait until after you have broken your fast to get started.

While you are fasting, you are still allowed to consume water, coffee and tea as long as you don't add anything with calories into them. If you know you are going to be pushing up against the 16 hour limit then you may want to add some coconut oil and grass-fed butter to your coffee. This approach to fasting tells your body that it is time for the cells to burn fat to obtain energy and to clean house. Crescendo fasting is a game changer for women. It will additionally boost your fertility and attractiveness. Within a couple of weeks, you will note the following benefits;

- Radiant skin
- Healthy libido
- Shiny hair
- An energetic demeanor
- Appropriate body weight

If you are over the age of 40, or are more than a few pounds overweight, then you might want to consider adding grass-fed collagen to your coffee on your fasting days instead. Collagen can reset your leptin levels which will help combat hunger. During fasting days it is important to keep both your fructose and sugars levels to a minimum as this will help to optimize leptin levels in the body. You can also add it to simple warm water if you don't prefer coffee or tea.

Chapter 3: 4:3 and 5:2 Fasting

The 4:3 and 5:2 style of fasting is quite similar to the Crescendo style of fasting except with more stringent caloric requirements all around. Y=The baseline caloric intake goal you should shoot for during either four of five days out of the week will be 2,000, and on the remaining days, you only consume somewhere between 500 and 600 calories. This is the favorite diet of actress Jennifer Aniston. The goal here is to ensure you don't feel deprived on the days that you are free to eat as you will while at the same time making sure that you don't do anything that would cause you to go overboard and ruin all of your hard work.

Studies surrounding this type of intermittent fasting show that it is likely to lead to an increased insulin resistance for those with diabetes, reduce the risk of heart arrhythmia, reduction of hot flashes and relief from both seasonal allergies and asthma. Additionally, a 12-week study of those using the 4:3 method revealed that the average practitioner saw a reduce in fat mass by 3.5 kg with no negative impact to muscle mass and an overall body weight reduction of 5 kg which came along with a 20 percent reduction in triglycerides and overall lower levels of blood pressure.

Perhaps most impressive, those who follow this type of intermittent fasting tend to see up to 40 percent lower leptin levels than normal. Additionally, they saw reduced levels of CRP which is a maker that indicates overall levels of inflammation in the body.

4:3 versus 5:2

The 4:3 plan is naturally more restrictive than the 5:2 plan simply because it allows you to eat less overall throughout the week. As such, you will need to more closely limit the amount of processed, refined or sugary foods that you consume on the days you do eat a full meal because it is likely that your body will crave these things, at least until you have thoroughly purged them from your diet.

As with all types of intermittent fasting, it is extremely important to avoid overindulging on the days that you are eating freely as it is extremely easy to eat 500 to 600 calories without even realizing it. If you keep it up, however, you will eventually be able to train your body to expect a diet that is more well-structured to ensure that you don't feel as hungry on your fast days. Think carefully about the foods you eat on these days as 500 calories can either be a handful of Oreos or a lightly seasoned fish filet and one will help you make it through far more easily than the other.

The 4:3 plan also recommends that you skip breakfast and measure your weight daily. For those whose weight tends to fluctuate more than average this is not recommended, however, as it can be disheartening without actually proving much one way or the other. If you do insist on going down this path, then you will need to be sure that you write your weight down every day and then average it out at the end of the week in order to get a true idea of where you are currently at.

Tips for success

Mix and match meal times: You have likely been eating at the same time each day (more or less) for so long at this point that you don't even think about mixing things up somewhat. However, not that you are changing up your overall eating schedule, it only makes sense to reevaluate what the best times to eat for you really are. On the days where you are only able to eat between 500 and 600 calories, you are likely going to want to wait as long as possible before you have your first meal as you are likely going to be less hungry in the morning anyway.

Likewise, rather than eating three 200 calorie snacks, you may only want to split your total in half instead. You will be surprised at how much fuller you are after 300 calories when compared to 200. The schedule that works for many people is 300 calories around noon and then the rest around 7 pm.

Minimize calories but maximize flavor: Soups are a great way to extend your caloric intake out as much as possible. Research into this type of fasting has shown that a vegetable soup can keep you feeling fuller for up to two extra hours compared to consuming the same number of calories purely through the vegetables themselves. What's more, with a soup you can go crazy on the seasonings, as long as they don't include carbs, which can help to trick your body into assuming that it has consumed something more substantial than 300 calories of soup. A good meal compensation for these days is two meals comprised primarily of vegetables with a small serving of protein such as tofu, lean meat, eggs or fish.

Stick with variety: When planning out your 500 and 600 calorie meals, it is important to try and stick with as many seasonal products as possible as this will help to ensure that your diet maintains a steady amount of variety and help to keep you healthy to boot. During the winter months, parsnips and butternut squash are great choices especially roasted or in a soup with some fetta cheese. If you are feeling up to a taste challenge, you can try some peppers (red or green) that have been cut in half and stuffed with tuna cream cheese or eggs and then grilled.

Additional foods for fasting day that you are sure to enjoy will include things like natural yogurt with berries, grilled fish, miso soup, tomato soup, cauliflower and backed eggs. When it comes to beverages you are going to want to stick exclusively to black coffee, tea and water. Coffee and tea are both natural appetite suppressants while also being a diuretic. If you lead a busy lifestyle then you can cheat with something prepackaged now and then but you should make every effort to stay away from them on a more regular basis.

Sample meal plan

Breakfast: Skip it. If you enjoy a morning meal then you will need to eliminate the snack during the day. You may also skip lunch instead.

Lunch: Lentil, leek or chicken soup with a small snack such as a tangerine.

Dinner: A small portion of fish or fillet of grilled chicken with a side salad with lemon juice and seasonings as dressing.

Snack: Carrot sticks to fill out the remainder of your calories.

Chapter 4: Eat-Stop-Eat Fasting

With this type of intermittent fasting, you can east normally 5 days a week before then fasting for as much as 24 hours on the other days of the week. It is important for women to only sprinkle this type of more extreme fasting into a more moderate type of fasting as it can cause hormonal imbalances if used to regularly.

When you are fasting, you will want to limit yourself to gum, water, coffee, tea and diet soda. You are also allowed small amounts of sugar-free cranberry juice. You can also consume bone broth in moderation as well, as long as you spread it out throughout the day. Ice pops are another useful way to help fight off hunger pains as well. On the days you are eating you can more or less eat what you will, assuming you don't use this as an excuse to ruin all of your hard work. You should make an effort to eat as many fresh fruits and vegetables as possible during this time in order to ensure your body is getting enough nutrients to see you through your fasting days as well.

Furthermore, you are going to want to up your daily protein intake to around 200 grams of protein per day, especially if you are planning ton continue exercising while fasting. This works out to about 50 grams every three to four hours which means you will likely want to invest in a high-quality protein powder to ensure you can hit this goal. If you feel as though you still aren't losing weight reliably after practicing some type of intermittent fasting for at least a month then you may need to cut more carbohydrates out of your diet.

Without a doubt, this is definitely one of the more extreme types of intermittent fasting and the simple truth is that going without eating for a full 24 hours will simply not be for everyone. You will know that you should look elsewhere for intermittent fasting options if you cannot make it through a 24 hour fast without experiencing headaches and dizziness for extended periods, even after your body has otherwise adapted to the intermittent fasting lifestyle. With that being said, the benefits of this intermittent fasting method are undeniable and it offers the freedom to alter when you are fasting based on need. Whatever you do, however, it is important to never fast for 2 consecutive days and never fast for more than 2 days in a single week.

Maintain your hydration: While this method of intermittent fasting is extremely strict, it is vital that you remain hydrated during this time to ensure you don't actually end up doing more harm than good. This is important as not only will it allow you to more easily deal with the lack of food but it will also help you remain hydrated as being in a fasted state is naturally dehydrating.

Further suggestions: When utilizing this or any of the other more extreme forms of intermittent fasting it is vital that you maintain your self-control when you first break your fast as going from zero to 60 with your food consumption could potentially damage your body and your fast will end up doing more harm than good. If you fall into a cycle of bingeing and purging then your system will likely end up in havoc and you may actually end up gaining weight no matter how little you are actually eating. As such, it is important to take a look inside and be honest with yourself when it comes to considering your overall level of self-control. If you have anything less than an iron will when it comes to food, then this might not be the type of intermittent fasting for you.

On those days when you are not actively fasting, you will want to pepper in resistance-style weight training to boost your overall results even more. On the days you are fasting you are going to want to take it very easy as if you overdue it, you are going to end up paying for it for quite some time. This means you are going to want to add in some yoga or light cardio but anything more is asking for trouble. Remember, forcing yourself through a tough workout on your fasting days isn't a feat of endurance that is going to be rewarded, it is essentially self-flagellation and all it is going to do is burn through what little energy your body was hanging onto to keep itself going, making the rest of your fast much more difficult in the process.

During the early days of your experience with this type of intermittent fasting, it is perfectly natural for you to feel anxious, angry or fatigued while also experiencing headaches and light-headedness. Remember, these symptoms should fade once your body gets used to this type of fasting if they don't discontinue using it ASAP and also consult a healthcare professional.

Chapter 5: Leangains Fasting

This type of intermittent fasting requires that women fast every day for 14 hours while then eating a reasonable amount throughout the rest of the day. This type of intermittent fasting has been shown to lead to the most noticeable weight loss in the overall shortest period of time. What's more, proponents of this type of fasting are quick to point out that you are likely to be asleep for at least half of the time you will be fasting, assuming you want to be, which makes this type of fasting far more manageable than it might seem on its face.

During the period of time during the day when you are not fasting you can then break your calorie count up any way you like as long as you are still cutting out about 500 calories per day while being conscious of what you are eating for the rest of the day. When you are fasting, you will want to limit yourself to just the basics, diet soda, black coffee, tea and water. For the best results for those who are either already overweight or have a mainly sedimentary lifestyle, cutting out most, if not all, starchy carbs from your diet is also recommended.

At first, you may find it difficult to fit the sum total of your caloric requirements into the limited window, but you will find that it gets easier with time as your body adjusts to the new eating timeframe. Most people who are following this type of fasting plan end up either eating two large meals or three regular-sized meals closer together and you are encouraged to try both and see which works better for you. Whichever direction you end up going, it is important to keep in mind the fact that consistency is the key to long-term success.

A recent study performed by the Obesity Society found that the most effective time to fast is going to be between 12 am and 2 pm. In fact, if you wait until 2 pm to have your first meal you will find that you reduce your overall feelings of hunger for the rest of the day while also ensuring that you are able to burn as much fat as possible.

Of all the various types of intermittent fasting, odds are you will find that this is the one that can be most easily adapted to fit your person schedule, whatever that may be. What's more, as long as you manage to get all your calories packed into the given amount of time, there is no reason that you should be able to go without until 2 pm comes around again. The most common eating pattern of followers of this type of intermittent fasting is to eat at 2 pm and then again around 8 pm with a large dinner that will then tide them over throughout the next day. This will ensure you can eat at relatively normal times that can fit into most schedules without too much effort. Regardless, you are ultimately free to break your schedule up in any way that works for you.

If you find that you are having a hard time getting started on or sticking with the Leangains form of intermittent fasting then it may be due to the fact that you are working too hard to forcing a schedule that doesn't naturally work for you. Make a breakdown of your average week and see what period of time would be easiest for you to go without for 14 hours. Once you do find this timeframe, you will then want to strive to lock it in as quickly as possible in order to make the transition as painless as can be expected on your body.

If you find that the final few hours of your fast seem to be a serious struggle no matter what you try to do, then the odds are good that you are not consuming enough protein throughout the day. You are going to want to aim for a minimum of 60 grams per day, or more if you are exercising. If you feel as though your protein intake is on point, then try looking into some options that are high in healthy fats as these will help tide you over as well.

This type of intermittent fasting is ideal for those who plan on exercising while fasting as it means you will still be consuming enough food every day to not really have to worry about holding back on your existing exercise routine as long as you take it easy during the transition period. If you plan on truly giving it your all then you are going to want to work to always break your fast with lots of dark green leafy vegetables, nuts, and seeds. When these are consumed in tandem they combine to give you a serious shot of energy and the protein you will need to make it through the day. Keeping your energy levels up throughout a fast can be though but if you make it a focus then you should be able to find something that works for you without too much trouble.

Generally speaking, your best choice is going to be breaking your fast with an average meal before exercising within the next four hours and then eating another larger meal as soon as you are finished with your workout. During this larger meal, you will want to focus on consuming enough complex carbohydrates to power yourself through the next day. By making a concentrated effort to fuel up fully, you will be able to make Leangains a part of your life in the long-term.

If you do not plan on exercising quite so much when on the Lean gains plan, then you will want to add in additional healthy fats instead of protein. If you are aiming to lose more than 20 pounds, then you will need to watch what you are eating carefully in order to ensure that you are bringing in at least .7 grams of healthy fat per pound of body weight in order to see the best results. Regardless, you should go out of your way to avoid simple carbs, unhealthy fats and processed foods and focus on natural alternatives whenever possible.

If you plan on mixing in some exercise into your intermittent fasting plan, then you will need to be sure to run the numbers for both types of days and eat accordingly in order to ensure you don't accidentally overeat. On the days you don't plan to exercise, you will want to ensure you maintain your weight loss by consuming 60 percent of your daily calories during the first mean and the rest in the second meal, and switch this if you plan to exercise.

Chapter 6: Alternative Types of Intermittent Fasting

Forever fat loss

This type of intermittent fasting is unique in that it combines various facets of several unique plans to form something all its own, what's especially neat is that it even comes with a weekly cheat day like you would see in many more traditional diets. To balance out this cheat day, however, you are then not allowed to consume anything except the bare minimum of what is allowed during a 24 hour fast for a full 36 hours which means this is not going to be a fast that you want to stick with in the long-term. You are also allowed a serving of dark, leafy green vegetables after 18 hours. For the rest of the week, you then follow the Leangains fasting schedule.

Fasting for 36 hours is naturally going to put this type of fasting out of the range of all but the most dedicated intermittent fasters, and even then, it is clearly an advanced technique as it is pushing up against the limits of what a person can safely manage. Additionally, the variety in the days means you are likely going to need a schedule that is somewhat flexible in order to account for the differences. Finally, you are going to need to limit any strenuous activity during your long fast if you ever hope to make it through successfully.

When you make it to the end of the long fast you will want to avoid eating too much too soon as it will be very easy to go overboard if you don't have absolute control. Starting with a small meal is vital to ensure that your digestive processes have time to spin back up before you get to the main course. If you feel as though you are having difficulty controlling yourself during the fast, or if you feel as though you need to eat as much as possible as soon as you break the fast then this is likely not going to be the right choice for you in the long-term. Your goal when fasting, regardless of the type of fasting it may be, is to find a solution that remains a healthy and sustainable choice in the long-term. Part of this means understanding that if a part of a specific plan ends up causing you to act in a way that is even remotely unhealthy then you will need to check yourself or choose a different method.

With that being said, if you can manage it, the results from this style of intermittent fasting make even the Leangains method pale in comparison. If you plan on following through with this type of intermittent fasting, then it is vital that you take extra care and ensure that your nutritional and caloric intake don't drop below normal. Additionally, before you attempt this plan then it is crucial you first consult a healthcare professional.

Alternate fasting
If you don't feel as though you can go a full 12 hours without almost passing out from hunger,

then you may find the alternate fasting method to be a better fit. With this style of intermittent fasting, you simply eat normally half of the time and then during the other half you cut your total intake to just 20 percent of your daily total. This will allow you to generate the same 3,500 calorie defect per week.

The downside to this fasting alternative is that you won't receive all of the benefits that come along with entering a fasted state. It is still a great place to start, however, as limiting your calories will help you to start to get in the habit of moderating your weighting and restricting your diet, while also putting you in a place where you can make additional positive choices more easily in the future.

If you are unsure of just how many calories you are consuming in a given day, it is important to always err on the side of consuming less than consuming more as hitting this 20 percent is key to seeing weight loss results. With that being said, it is important to determine the right number of calories for you as eating too few will lead to malnutrition scenarios which can ultimately lead to lasting bodily damage.

During your low-calorie days, you will want to do everything in your power to stretch those calories as far as they will going. One great choice when doing so is to use a protein powder as protein shakes are a great way to fill yourself up without sacrificing too many calories in the process. This should only be your plan to start, however, as a whole, natural foods are always going to be the better long-term choice.

This is actually one of the most popular types of fasting and those who couldn't deal with one of the more extreme options tended to be able to stick to it compared to other variations two to one. What's more the average weight loss during the transitional phase with this type of fasting is three pounds per week.

Irregular fasting

If you like the idea behind intermittent fasting but don't feel as though you are yet ready to commit to anything quite so permanent, then you may instead want to begin by simply fasting for at least 12 hours now and then, just to see what it is like. While this won't necessarily provide you with the full range of benefits you would get from committing more thoroughly to the process, it will still give you a pretty good idea of what to expect and if your body can easily handle the process of going without food for that length of time.

The key to success in this scenario is going to be to avoid thinking about it as an either-or proposition and instead take pride in the fact that you are doing more than the bare minimum of what can be done in your current situation. Anything that can be done in order makes you even a little bit healthier is never going to be the wrong choice. What's more, each time you fast you will make it a little bit easier as you start to develop the physical and mental determination to pick up the process in the long-term. It doesn't matter how long it takes or if you start and stop repeatedly before making the switch, the only thing you have to lose from the process is unwanted weight.

Chapter 7: Exercise and Intermittent Fasting

While intermittent fasting can provide you with a wide variety of benefits when it comes to increased weight loss and increased muscle mass, if you want to really kick things into high gear then you will want to ensure that you are exercising regularly throughout as well. What exercise while fasting looks like is going to largely depend on you and what your exercise plan looked like before you started intermittent fasting. It will also depend on which type of fasting you are attempting and ultimately how your body responds to adding exercise into your fasting process.

Adding exercise to your intermittent fasting plan

The food you eat is directly responsible for the amount of fuel that your body has to power itself and build new muscle while it is exercising. As such, it isn't too much of a leap to understand that when you aren't eating you are naturally going to have a more difficult time exercising and see fewer results as well. It doesn't matter if you are working on strength or endurance training, your body mainly uses glycogen which is extracted from the carbohydrates that you eat in order to provide you the energy you need to exercise at maximum efficiency.

Nevertheless, if your glycogen reserves are running low, such as when you are getting close to the end of your fast, then your body is going to need to look for other sources of energy to power its exercise routine. As such, once your body has gotten used to doing so, you will find that you burn as much as 20 percent fatter if you exercise right before you finish your fast as opposed to right before you get started.

Unfortunately, this isn't only good news as if glycogen is in limited supply then your body is likely to burn some protein in addition to fat, in order to ensure your bodily process are working as intended. Due to the fact that protein is also responsible for creating healthy muscles, if you fail to take the right precautions then you could end up dropping fat and muscle while you are fasting. This will do more than just affect how much you can bench press or how toned your body looks, it will also slow down your metabolism which can make it difficult for you to lose weight in the long run once your body adapts to the number of calories you are now consuming on a regular basis.

This means that once your body adapts to its new routine you will naturally have more energy left over for things like exercise in addition to all of your core bodily functions. You can expect it to take about a month for your body to fully adapt to the process. When it comes to merging your existing exercise plan with intermittent fasting, it is vital that you keep in mind that all types of exercise are going to be more difficult right off the bat than what you may remember.

This is perfectly natural, of course, you are exercising on an empty stomach after all. Due to the fact that your blood sugar levels and glycogen levels are going to be lower than normal as well, you will likely feel weaker to start to boot. This means it is extremely important to schedule your workout at the appropriate time depending on the goals you have set for yourself. Just make sure you are giving your body the tools it needs to take advantage of all of your hard work.

Exercise tips

Stick with low intensity exercises: If you plan on exercising regularly while fasting, it is crucial that you limit your cardio to only that of the low intensity variety. This means you will want to avoid doing anything that you can't carry on a normal conversation during the midst of. This equates to things such as a light jog or 10 minutes on the stationary bike, as long as you aren't pushing yourself past your limits.

It is going to be extremely important to take the time to listen to the signals your body is giving you and to immediately take a break if you feel as though you are starting to get light-headed or dizzy as both of these conditions are going to appear far more frequently than they otherwise would. If you ignore what your body is trying to tell you and attempt to power through, then it is only going to make the rest of your workout seem all that more unmanageable.

Timing is key: This is not to say that you want to avoid pushing yourself while fasting, far from it, instead it is about choosing the right times to do so in order to ensure the best overall results. The best times to take on an extremely strenuous workout is going to be roughly an hour after you've broken your fast. This will allow your body to get some energy into your system before you start exercising and pushing things to the limit.

Plan more: When it comes to weight loss, it is important that you exercise on an empty stomach. While fasting you won't want to keep things at a strenuous pace, and instead, consider going for an early morning jog or a low-intensity spin class. Even if you are keeping it light, however, if you are planning to exercise with several hours of fasting left to go then you need to ensure that your dinner is going to leave you with enough energy to do what you need to do without being miserable afterwards.

If you are planning on doing a cardio workout in the morning, for example, then you are going to want to ensure you have built up your glycogen stores using complex carbohydrates the night before. While it is important to have the fuel you need, you should make it a point to never exercise on a full stomach. The most important thing to keep in mind is to plan ahead to ensure that your nutrition needs, and your exercise needs are well matched, even if you exercise first thing in the morning or late at night.

Choose the right approach: Generally speaking, there is no upper limit as to the amount of exercise you can do while you are fasting, as long as you listen to what your body is telling you and not pushing yourself so hard that you are doing yourself harm, keep up the good work. In fact, some studies even suggest that strength increases right up to the 16 hours mark which fasting. With that being said, it is important to always take things slow at first, it is much easier to amp things up then it is to recover from an injury that only occurred because you went too hard too fast.

If you are looking to go as hard as possible, fasting or no fasting, then you are going to want to focus on adding more protein to your diet to ensure your body has the tools it needs to keep building your muscles. If you keep things as carb focused as the Standard American Diet likes then you will find yourself regularly running out of fuel and starting to feel weak, nauseous, lightheaded, and dizzy. Feeling weak and nauseous is a surefire indicator that your glycogen levels are depleted, something you don't want to happen if you aren't in sight of your next eating period. Finding the right mixture of exercise that strengthens the muscles without pushing them to the limit and burning the maximum amount of fat possible.

Sports nutritionists suggest working out during your feeding window. If you work out during your feeding window, you will be able to have your meal immediately after an intense workout session. You will also be able to enjoy a healthy snack before your workouts. Think about exercises such as taking a brisk 20 to 30-minute walk in the park or around your neighborhood, which is not as intensive as the sweat sessions you may be used to. If you prefer working out in the morning, then you can reschedule your eating window to the 8.00 am - 4.00 pm window. This will shift your fasting hours so that you begin at 4.00 pm until the following morning.

Cardio: Studies show that if you are looking for a great way to burn as much fat as possible while fasting, then the best way to go about doing so is by going hard on the cardio first on the days that you aren't fasting, and then on the days that you are as well. It also decreases bad cholesterol and promotes good cholesterol at the same time.

Recommended cardio exercises with intermittent fasting for weight loss include;

- Cycling
- Running
- Jumping rope
- High intensity interval training is another great choice as it involves repeating a number of exercises in short bursts. If you are looking to maximize your workouts in a

minimum amount of time, then this is a great place to start.

Weight training: When it comes to weight training successfully while maintaining an intermittent fasting lifestyle, the most important thing to keep in mind is to keep your overall protein consumptions as high as possible to ensure you have plenty of key muscle building blocks left over for your fasting days as well. Even still, you are going to want to take it much easier on your fasting days as your body is already running on fumes as it is. Early on you may want to start with only cardio on your fasting days and strength training on your non-fast days until your body adapts to the difference in lifestyle before adding in some light strength training on the fasting days.

One of the key protocols of successful weightlifting routines is to keep your training sessions as focused and intense as possible. Think of strategies such as the reverse pyramid. This is a training strategy for muscle gain and massive strength. This type of strategy requires that you start with the heaviest set first. It means doing the heaviest work when you are still fresh and fully capable. With each set, you become fatigued with lower energy levels. The best part of this strategy is that you can give your all in the first set knowing that you won't need to replicate it again. This makes it so easy to progress.

It is important to always exercise with a clear plan in mind, and to also track the workouts you do complete to track your progress and keep everything on track. On those days where you don't quite feel up to exercising then you can simply look back at all the hard work you have already done in order to find the mental fortitude to carry on.

Focus on nutritious post-work out snacks: Generally speaking, you will feel better overall if you can eat before and after you exercise to ensure your body has all the fuel it needs and that you can get back all the energy you exerted without waiting hours to refuel. Nuts are a great post-work out snack that can keep you going until you can find something more substantial to put into your body.

Healthy Recipes

The following list of recipes are either high in protein, healthy fats, carbs, or some combination of the three, they are great examples of the types of meals you should shoot for when exercising regularly while intermittent fasting as they will ensure you have the fuel you need to go the distance.

Chicken enchilada

This recipe needs 30 minutes of active preparation, 15 minutes of cooking time and will serve 6.

- Protein: 43 grams
- Net Carbs: 7 grams
- Fats: 28 grams
- Calories: 447

What to Use

- Salt (as desired)
- Pepper (as desired)
- Coconut oil (2 T)
- Cheddar cheese (2 c)
- Green chilies (4 oz. chopped)
- Queso fresco (1 c)
- Chicken breasts (1 lb.)
- Enchilada sauce (1.5 c)

What to Do

- Start by making sure your oven is heated to 450F.

- Pat the chicken to ensure it is dry before mixing together the salt and pepper in a small bowl and using the results to coat the chicken thoroughly.

- Place the chicken in a saucepan along with the enchilada sauce before placing the pan on the stove on top of a burner turned to a low/medium heat and let it simmer, covered, for 10 minutes before flipping the chicken and letting it simmer for another 10 minutes or until it has reached an internal temperature of 165 degrees check the temperature using a meat thermometer.

- Let the chicken cool before shredding it into bite-sized pieces using a pair of forks and placing it in a mixing bowl. Add in the chilies, queso fresco and enchilada sauce and mix well. Season as needed.

- Prepare a baking dish by coating it in oil before spreading 1 c cheese on the base of the dish before adding in the chicken mixture and topping with the remaining cheese.

- Cover the dish in foil before placing it in the oven for approximately 10 minutes. Remove the foil and return it to the oven for 3 more minutes to give the cheese plenty of time to melt.

Zucchini nachos

This recipe needs 15 minutes of active preparation, 20 minutes of cooking time and will serve 4.

- Protein: 44 grams
- Net Carbs: 6.3 grams
- Fats: 38.6 grams
- Calories: 578

What to Use - Meat

- Oregano leaves (.25 tsp.)
- Red pepper flakes (.25 tsp.)
- Onion powder (.25 tsp.)
- Garlic powder (.25 tsp.)
- Cumin (.5 tsp. ground)
- Paprika (.5 tsp.)
- Chili powder (.5 T)
- Ground beef (.5 lbs.)
- Coconut oil (2 T)

What to Use – Guacamole

- Vitamin C crystals (1 pinch)
- Salt (.25 tsp.)

- Oregano (.5 tsp. dried)
- Apple cider vinegar (1 T)
- MCT Oil (1 T)
- Vital proteins collagen peptides (2 T)
- Avocado (1)

What to Use – The Rest
- Green onion (2 sliced)
- Mexican cheese blend (.5 c)
- Zucchini (2 sliced into rounds)

What to Do
- Cover a serving plate with parchment paper before placing the zucchini onto it in such a way that it does not overlap, you will likely have to cook it in batches.
- Place the plate in the microwave and let the zucchini cook for 8 minutes on 50 percent power. You will know they are ready when the edges begin to curl upwards. Place the cooked zucchini onto a cooling rack.

- Add the oil to a pan before placing the pan on the stove over a burner turned to a medium heat. Add in the meat, along with all of the relevant seasonings and brown the meat thoroughly.
- Add all of the ingredients for the guacamole to a bowl and mash thoroughly.
- Place the zucchini chips back onto the serving plate, add the meat on top, followed by the guacamole and top with additional cheese prior to serving.

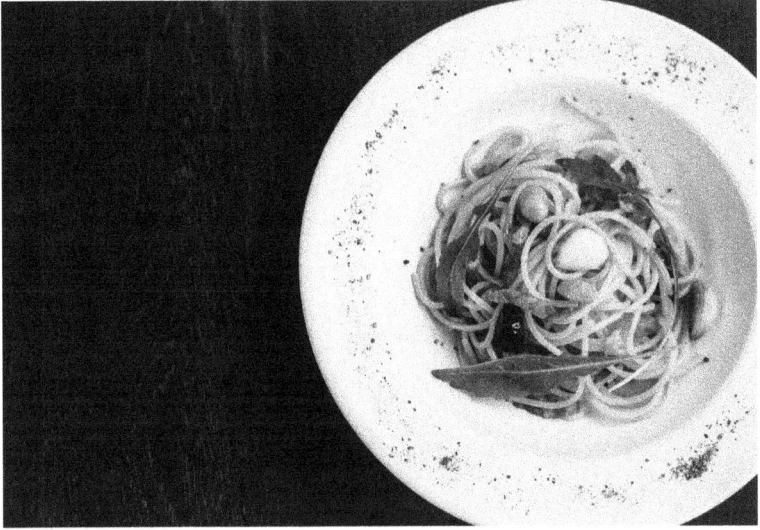

Grecian Chicken Pasta

This recipe needs 15 minutes to prepare, 15 minutes to cook and will make 6 servings.

- Protein: 42.6 grams
- Carbs: 70 grams
- Fats: 11.4 grams
- Calories: 488

What to Use

- Olive oil (1 T)
- Red onion (.5 c chopped)
- Linguine (16 oz.)

- Pepper (as desired)
- Salt (as desired)
- Lemons (2 wedged)
- Oregano (2 tsp. dried)
- Lemon juice (2 T)
- Parsley (3 T chopped)
- Feta cheese (.5 c crumbled)
- Tomato (1 chopped)
- Marinated artichoke hearts (14 oz. chopped, drained)
- Chicken breast (1 lb. cubed)
- Garlic (2 cloves crushed)

What to Do

- Fill a large pot with water and a pinch of salt before placing it on the stove on top of a burner that has been turned to a high heat. Once the water boils, add in the pasta and let it cook until it is still firm but just starting to become tender, which should take approximately 8 minutes.

- Add the olive oil to a skillet before placing it on top of a burner turned to a high/medium heat. Place the garlic and onion into the skillet and let it cook for approximately 2 minutes until it begins to be fragrant.

- Mix in the chicken and stir regularly until the chicken ceases to be pink and all of its juices are clear, this should take approximately 5 minutes. The chicken should end up with an internal temperature of 165F.

- Turn the burner to a low/medium heat before adding in the pasta, oregano, lemon juice, parsley, feta cheese, tomato and artichoke hearts. Let the results cook while stirring for roughly 2 minutes.

- Remove the skillet from the burner, season as desired and garnish using the lemon prior to serving.

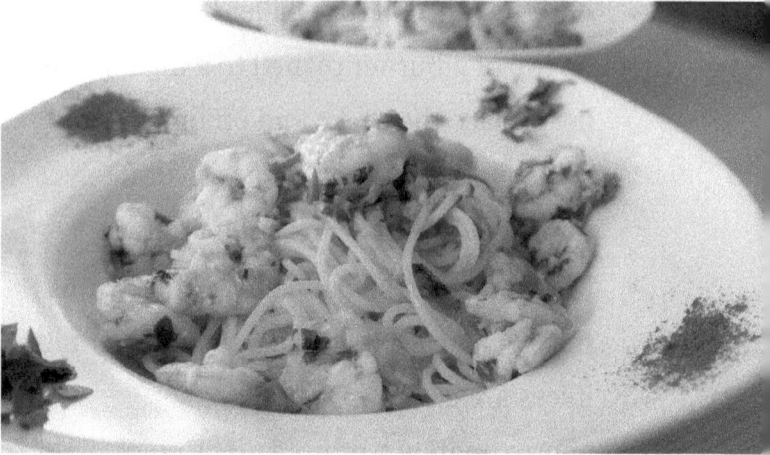

Shrimp and Penne

This recipe needs 10 minutes to prepare, 20 minutes to cook and will make 8 servings.

- Protein: 34.5 grams
- Carbs: 48.5 grams
- Fats: 8.5 grams
- Calories: 385

What to Use

- Pepper (as desired)
- Salt (as desired)
- Extra virgin olive oil (2 T)

- Parmesan cheese (1 c grated)
- Shrimp (1 lb. deveined, peeled)
- Tomatoes (29 oz. diced)
- White wine (.25 c)
- Garlic (1 T chopped)
- Red onion (.25 c)
- Olive oil (2 T)
- Penne pasta (16 oz.)

What to Do

- Fill a large pot with water and a pinch of salt before placing it on the stove on top of a burner that has been turned to a high heat. Once the water boils, add in the pasta and let it cook for about 8 minutes until it reaches an al dente state.
- Add the olive oil to a skillet before placing it on top of a burner turned to a high/medium heat. Place the garlic and onion into the skillet and cook until the onion begins to turn tender. Add in the wine along with the

tomatoes and let everything cook for 10 minutes, stirring regularly.

- Add in the shrimp and let it cook for 5 minutes. Toss with the pasta and top with parmesan cheese prior to serving.

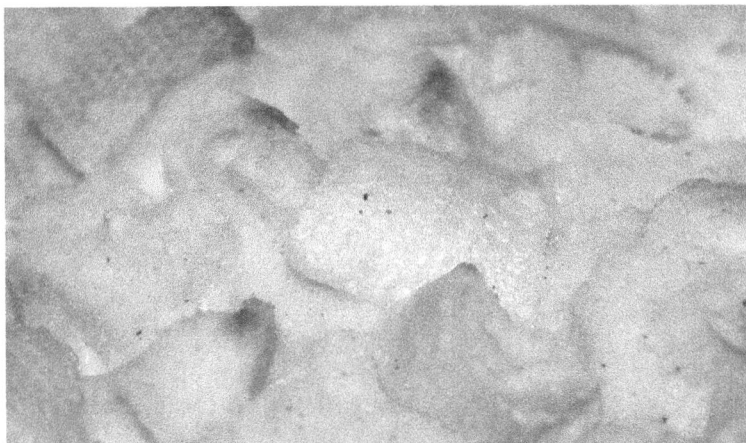

Bread Pudding

This recipe needs 30 minutes of preparation, 15 minutes of cooking time and will serve 2.

- Protein: 60.4 grams
- Carbs: 20.4 grams
- Fiber: 20.7 grams
- Sugar: 3.5 grams
- Fats: 3.5 grams
- Calories: 300

What to use

- Egg yolk (1)
- Maple syrup (1 T)

- Organic vanilla extract (.25 T)
- Egg (1)
- Coconut milk (.5 c)
- Grain free bread (4 slices)

What to Do

- Line a pot that will fit inside the Instant Pot cooker pot, using parchment paper.
- Add the vanilla, syrup, yolk, egg and milk into a blender and blend for 10 seconds before adding in the melted unsalted butter.
- Add water to the Instant Pot cooker pot before adding in a trivet and placing the line pot on top of it before adding in the bread to the pot on top of the trivet.
- Add the results from the blender to the top pot, taking care to press on the bread to distribute the mixture evenly.
- Place a small parchment square over the pudding.
- Place the Instant Pot cooker pot into the Instant Pot cooker and seal the lid. Choose

the steam option and set the time for 15 minutes.

- Once the timer goes off, select the natural pressure release option and allow the pot to sit for 20 minutes.
- Allow the Instant Pot cooker to cool for 5 minutes before using the parchment paper to remove the pudding.
- Transfer the pudding to a serving dish and flip prior to serving.

Chuck roast

This recipe needs 25 minutes of preparation, 180 minutes of cooking time and will serve 2.

- Protein: 49 grams
- Carbs: 50.1 grams
- Fiber: 44.8 grams
- Sugar: 9.7 grams
- Fats: 22.3 grams
- Calories: 620

What to use

- Garlic powder (.25 tsp.)
- Unsalted butter (3 T melted)
- Vegetable oil (.25 t)
- Bay leaf (.5 dried)
- Low-sodium beef broth (14 oz.)
- Red wine (.5 c)
- Garlic powder (.5 tsp.)
- Onion (.25 sliced)
- Black pepper (as desired)
- Chuck roast (1 lb.)

What to Do

- Combine the seasonings together in a small bowl and season the roast as desired, allow it to sit at room temperature for about 20 minutes.

- Add the oil to the Instant Pot cooker pot and place it into the Instant Pot cooker before setting the heat to sauté and adding in the meat, allowing it to flame roast on all sides.

- Add in the onions and allow them to cook for 5 minutes until they are soft and brown. Add in the red wine and allow it to simmer until it has reduced 50 percent. Make sure to scrape the bottom of the pan while allowing it to simmer.

- Add in the bay leaf and beef broth before returning the roast back to the pot and sealing the lid. Choose the stew/meat option and set the time for 100 minutes.

- Once the timer goes off, select the natural pressure release option and allow the pot to sit for 25 minutes before venting the excess pressure.

- Remove the roast to the serving tray before running the resulting liquid through a strainer and using it to top meat prior to serving.

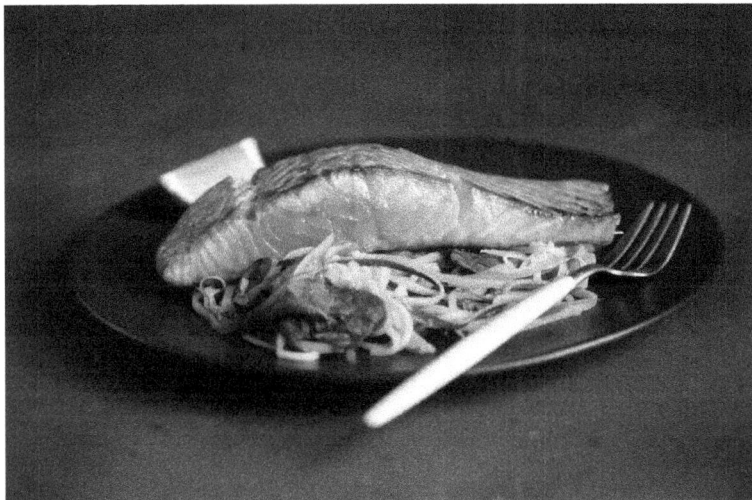

Pesto Salmon with Spinach

This recipe needs 17 minutes to prepare and will make 2 servings.

- Protein: 32 grams
- Net Carbs: 9 grams
- Fats: 53 grams
- Calories: 671

What to Use

- Coconut Oil (1 teaspoon)
- Crushed Walnuts (0.5 cups)
- Spinach (10 oz)

- Pesto (0.5 cup)
- Garlic (2 teaspoons)
- Salmon (2 filets)

What to Do

- Ensure your oven is preheated to 350 degrees Fahrenheit.
- Use coconut oil to lightly grease your baking dish. Sprinkle half of the total amount of spinach you have at the bottom.
- Lay salmon over spinach bed, and sprinkle with garlic.
- Gently spread pesto out over salmon.
- Cover entire dish with remaining spinach.
- Allow the mixture to cook for roughly 12 minutes, or until salmon is cooked through.

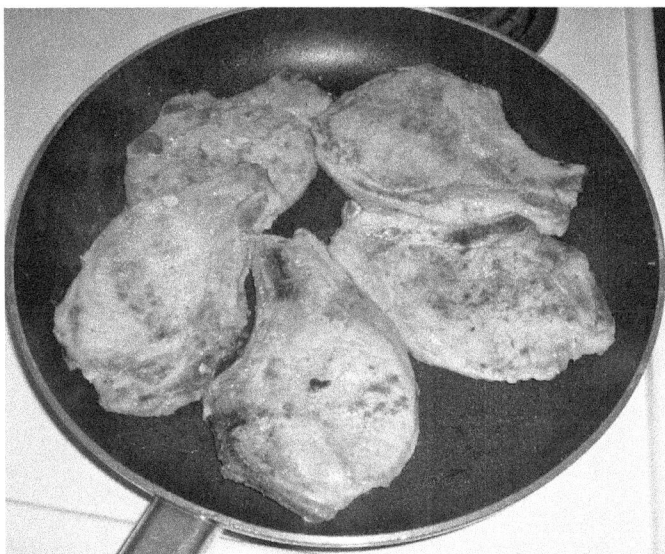

Blackened Pork Chops

This recipe needs 15 minutes to prepare and will make 4 servings.

- Protein: 46 grams
- Net Carbs: 4 grams
- Fats: 25 grams
- Calories: 341

What to Use

- Cumin (1 teaspoon ground)
- Butter (4 tablespoons)
- Thyme Leaves (0.5 teaspoons)

- Black Pepper (2 teaspoons)
- Cayenne Pepper (0.25 teaspoon)
- Garlic Powder (1 teaspoon)
- Onion Powder (1 teaspoon)
- Sea Salt (2 teaspoons)
- Paprika (1 tablespoon)
- Pork Chops (4 total)
- Oregano (0.5 teaspoons dried)

What to Do

- Blend spices in small bowl.
- Melt all of the butter in a separate bowl in the microwave.
- In a medium skillet, heat bacon grease until hot. Dip pork chops in melted butter, coat them with spice blend and then place in skillet with bacon grease.
- Cook for 5 minutes without touching, then flip and cook again for another 5 minutes. The internal temperature should reach 140-150 degrees Fahrenheit.
- Transfer pork chops to plate and serve with a desired side dish.

Bacon Burger

This recipe needs 10 minutes to prepare, 10 minutes to cook and will make 1 serving.

- Protein: 43.5 grams
- Net Carbs: 1.8 grams
- Fats: 51.8 grams
- Calories: 649

What to Use

- Worcestershire sauce (.25 tsp.)
- Onion powder (.25 tsp.)
- Salt (.5 tsp.)
- Soy sauce (.75 tsp.)
- Black pepper (.5 tsp.)
- Garlic (.5 tsp. minced)
- Chives (1.5 tsp. chopped)
- Cheddar cheese (2 T sliced)
- Bacon (2 slices cooked, chopped)
- Beef (9.5 oz. ground)

What to Do

- Place a skillet over a medium/high heat before adding in the chopped bacon and letting it cook until it reaches your desired level of crispness.
- After the bacon has finished cooking remove it from the pan but retain the grease for later use.
- Add 60 percent of the bacon, the ground beef, the Worcestershire sauce, onion powder, salt, soy sauce, chives, black pepper and garlic to a mixing bowl and mix well before forming the results into 3 patties.
- Add the bacon grease bacon into the skillet and place the skillet on a burner turned to a high heat. Let the patties cook for up to 5 minutes depending on the level of doneness that you prefer.
- Let the patties sit for 3 minutes and top with cheese prior to serving.

Cinnamon and Orange Beef Stew

This recipe needs 20 minutes to prepare, 3 hours to cook and will make 1 serving.

- Protein: 53.5 grams
- Net Carbs: 1.9 grams
- Fats: 44.5 grams
- Calories: 649

What to Use

- Bay leaf (1)
- Sage (.25 tsp.)
- Rosemary (.25 tsp.)
- Fish sauce (.5 tsp.)
- Soy sauce (.5 tsp.)
- Cinnamon (.5 tsp. ground)
- Garlic (.75 tsp. minced)
- Thyme (.75 tsp.)
- Orange (.25 juiced)
- Orange (.25 zest)
- Onion (.25 medium)
- Coconut oil (1 T)
- Beef broth (.75 cups)
- Beef (.5 lbs. cubed)

What to Do

- This recipe can easily be doubled or tripled if you want to set aside extra for leftovers.

- You are going to want to start by adding the coconut oil to your skillet before setting over a burned turned to a high heat and letting it reach the smoke point.

- Add in the meat in batches and season as desired. Let each batch of beef brown completely prior to moving on to the next batch of beef.

- After all of the beef has browned, add in the onion and garlic and let them cook for 1.5 minutes before adding in the orange juice, bay, fish sauce, orange zest, soy sauce, cinnamon and thyme.

- Let the results cook for 20 seconds before adding it all to the slow cooker along with the remaining seasonings.

- Cover your slow cooker and let it cook on a high heat for 1.5 hours.

Chapter 8: Tips for Success

While no one is questioning the fact that intermittent fasting is undeniably useful, that doesn't mean that it still can't be difficult to get started with or to get into enough of a habit to make it into a lifelong lifestyle change. As such, the following tips have been compiled as guideposts to help point you towards your ultimate success. Don't forget, intermittent fasting is a marathon, not a spring which means slow and steady is the only way to find the success you seek.

Know yourself: While there is no denying the health benefits associated with intermittent fasting, this doesn't mean that it is the right choice for you, right now. While anyone can make it through a few days of intermittent fasting, it is important to consider any external or internal factors that may make it difficult for you to keep it up for a full 30 days right now.

It takes about four weeks to form a new habit which means if you can't commit to that timeframe right now, then you might be putting yourself through a lot of undue stress for no particularly tangible reason. If everything in your life isn't going to align in such a way to make intermittent fasting a viable proposition for you, right now, then there is no shame in choosing a more opportune time to start.

Additionally, it is important to consider how disciplined you really are, what your relationship with food is like and how healthy you are overall in general. For example, if you have always eaten poorly and are now looking for a way to start down a healthier path, skipping right to the eat-stop-eat method is only going to lead to serious issues. First, you will find that you have a hard time sticking with the fast as you have never withheld food before. Second, you likely won't lose as much as you might otherwise as your body isn't used to being deprived of the food it wants when it wants it. Finally, you will end up feeling dejected about intermittent fasting in general and your ability to follow through specifically. Remember, it is a lot easier to be realistic about your chance of success and decide to look elsewhere before you get started in earnest than after struggling with and failing at fasting after a week or more of serious effort.

Listen to your body: Listening to what your body is telling you is a key part to successfully intermittently fasting in the long-term. However, this importance is at an all time high during the transitional period between when your body is still adjusting to the new way of eating. While it is perfectly normal to feel weak from time to time, angry, irritable, shaky, lightheaded or faint, if these symptoms become an everyday occurrence then it is a surefire sign that something isn't right. It is important to be in touch with your body enough to know when it is time to take a break from intermittent fasting and contact a healthcare professional.

Be realistic: While you are sure to see weight loss while your body is first adapting to consuming fewer calories on the regular, this is bound to eventually taper off as your body adjusts to work with what you are giving it. Additionally, it is perfectly natural for the weight loss to stop and start during the first month as your body tries to hang on to the calories it has while it tries to figure out just what is going on.

After it gets with the program, you should expect to maintain an average weight loss of about a pound a week as anything more than this is untenable for your body in the long run. Don't forget, it is perfectly natural to hit plateaus during any weight loss plan and the best way to get through them is to stay the course and let your body work itself out. The worst thing you can do if you hit a plateau is to try and change things up to get your weight loss back on track as this will only confuse your body and make it even more difficult for you to get things back on track.

Drink more water: More than 50 percent of adults are suffering from at least a mild degree of dehydration at any given time. As such, this piece of advice is extremely important as being in a fasted state is going to dehydrate you even more, which, when coupled with the lack of fuel in your system can turn a little bit of dizziness into a full-fledged fainting spell. While you are practicing intermittent fasting of any kind you should aim to drink a gallon of water each day.

Not only will this help you to feel fuller for longer once you have eaten, it will help your body to continue to process all of its toxins normally even if it is currently holding onto all of its fat because of the transition process. In fact, if you let your thirst go untreated for long enough, it actually starts to manifest as hunger so ensuring you remain properly hydrated is actually going to keep you feeling full in more ways than one.

Treat caffeine like a tool: While you are free to drink as much black coffee, tea or diet soda as you like, it is important to not rely on its hunger-curbing effects too heavily as it will make it difficult for your body to fully adjust to the process. Remember, once the transition has been made, your body will get used to this new way of eating and grow hungry accordingly. However, if you use large amounts of caffeine to curtail your appetite indefinitely then your body won't adapt to your new lifestyle and you will find yourself unable to truly progress in a meaningful way.

Additionally, while it is fine to hit the caffeine hard for the first week or so, it is important to avoid artificial sweeteners as much as possible as many of these have been known to cause health problems of their own if they are consumed in large amounts. Above all else, it is best that treat caffeine as you would any other chemical and only use it sparingly most of the time.

Stay busy: While your first instinct may be to attempt to hibernate as much as possible in order to get through the worst part of the transition period, the truth is this is just about the worst thing you can do. Freeing up your schedule on fast days is only going to remind you of how long you have to wait until you are able to eat again, making the hours between now and food seem interminable. As such, the better option is to instead pick a time to attempt the transition when you are extremely busy as then you will be able to blow through the hours when you aren't allowed to eat with ease.

Plan around your fast days: When it comes to successfully making intermittent fasting part of your long-term lifestyle, it is important to start thinking of your days based on when your mind and body are going to be at their peak when it comes to having the fuel they need to be their best. This means you should schedule the most arduous tasks of your day either first thing in the morning when you will naturally be less hungry anyway or about an hour after you have broken your fast which is when your reserve will be full once more.

Your body will naturally begin to slow down across the board, diverting what energy might be left to core bodily functions the further out it gets from a meal which means that difficult tasks will only get more difficult as the day goes on. Knowing what you're in for, and how to deal with it properly will make a big deal moving forward.

Don't let yourself make excuses: If you ever hope to successfully transition into an intermittent fasting lifestyle, it is extremely important that you understand that there will never be a perfect time to make any major lifestyle change. While there are certainly plenty of valid reasons to not start intermittent fasting tomorrow, when coming up with a timeframe to start it is important to not let valid reasons slide into excuse territory. For example, knowing you are going to be in recovery soon from surgery is a good reason to postpone starting intermittent fasting, having a busy schedule, not so much.

If you let it, your brain is always going to be able to come up with plausible sounding reasons to maintain its status quo. The only person who can ensure that you are actually motivated enough to make intermittent fasting work in your life is you. Committing to success and following through are the only ways to meet your weight loss goals, bar none.

Have realistic expectations: When starting your new intermittent fasting lifestyle, it is very important to not expect results overnight and to remember that a pound of fat lost per week is the average you should hope for. If you find yourself getting discouraged by your apparent lack of results early on, simply take the time to consider how long it took for you to reach your current weight and then cut yourself some slack. It is unreasonable to assume that something that took years to happen will be undone in weeks, or even months.

Try more than one type of fasting: When you first start practicing intermittent fasting, it can be easy to become infatuated with the first plan that you try that seems to generate visible results. While this plan could very well be a perfect fit for you, the fact of the matter is that without more plans to compare it to, you will have no real way of knowing if you are getting the most that you can from the process. There are plenty of different patterns of eating, with various frequency, size and number of meals which means it is important to not underestimate the importance of any one of these options. Mix and match a variety of fasting styles and times to see what your body responds to best.

Add BCAA to your diet: Branch chain amino acids are a very important supplement if you are planning to fast on a regular basis, especially if you are hoping to go beyond 14 hours. BCAA supplements will stimulate additional weight loss while at the same time ensuring that your lean muscle won't be broken down while your body looks for nutrients during your fast.

Start off slow: If you have never gone more than a few hours without eating before, then it is best that you start off slowly and work your way up to even the lightest intermittent fasting plan. You will likely be best served by starting at 10 hours without eating and building up your tolerance from there. Remember, intermittent fasting is a personal decision and you have no need to feel ashamed if it takes you longer to get started than it might for other people. Rather, you should feel proud that you are sticking with it despite the additional difficulties you are being forced to overcome. Once you begin to see real weight loss results you will notice that it will become easier to persevere, all you have to do is make it to that point and things will begin to fall into place.

Discretion is the better part of valor: While there is plenty of scientific evidence to support the ideas behind intermittent fasting, many people have a partial or flawed understanding of the process that can lead to some unfortunate confrontations if you aren't careful. While there is nothing wrong with a rational debate between two reasonable adults, you are likely to be on edge if you are still in the transitional period and likely unable to describe the finer points of the research which supports your new life choices. As such, it is often better to wait until you have made it through the rough patch and have plenty of personal evidence to draw from and until then, keep your new diet to yourself.

Don't be too hard on yourself: When you are first starting out, it is important to not only understand that the transitional period can be rough for some people but also to understand what that means for you. While it is certainly important to hold yourself accountable in order to ensure that you don't make poor choices in the long run, when you are first starting out there is no reason to be ashamed if you only make it 13 hours instead of 14. The transition period is going to be difficult enough with the very real physical issues you will be dealing with, you don't need to add additional mental stress to the mix as well.

As such, when you are first starting out there is no reason not to reward yourself when you make it through a full week without breaking your new patterns. Rewards will help your brain to establish new patterns more quickly and will also give you positive connotations to associate the process with, aiding your progress as well. As long as you don't let it get out of hand, there is no harm in having an extra decadent dessert, remember you only need to cut out 3,500 calories to lose a pound, as long as you make it up elsewhere there is no need to hold yourself to the highest standards right away. Instead, consider how successful you have already been and understand that your brain is likely to link intermittent fasting with a delayed reward which means it will be easier to persevere in the long run.

Add more protein to your diet: Even if you aren't planning on exercising when you are in the midst of the transitional phase, you will find that if you add some extra protein to your diet then you will find that making it through the last few hours of your fast becomes far more manageable than would otherwise be the case. Beyond just fish, poultry and red meat, nuts and beans are both a great source of protein. For a little extra boost that's a little less natural, there are a wide variety of protein bars, shakes and powders that are made from all-natural ingredients though unprocessed options are always going to be a better choice in the long run.

Stay away from junk food: While there is nothing in the intermittent fasting ethos that prevents junk food per say, it is important to get out of the habit of eating it regularly for several reasons. First and foremost, almost everything on the average fast food menu is deceptively high in calories and unless you are doing your homework before getting into the drive through the line then it can be very easy to make a poor choice and end up negating all of your hard work without realizing it.

What's worse, that type of food is often full of lots of fillers, carbohydrates and bad fats which means that it is unlikely it is going to stick to your ribs for the amount of time you need it to if you want to last through your next fast without going over your daily calorie allotment in the interim. Beyond that, however, you are already putting so much effort into improving how you eat and your overall relationship with food and odds are after a few months that junk food will naturally lose its allure. Focus on foods that are high in protein and healthy fats and you will feel more full and energetic for longer periods every time. You only have so much time you can eat each day, make it count.

Consider the source of your hunger: Depending on your previous relationship with hunger, you may find that stopping to ask yourself why it is you really feel hungry is always a useful step in the process. However, it will be especially important early on as you are almost guaranteed to find yourself feeling hungry at the same time as you would naturally eat breakfast lunch and dinner. While there is certainly going to be some amount of truth to that hunger, odds are it won't be nearly as much as you might think.

The habits that you stuck to previously are going to continue to stick around for most of the first month but by being aware of this fact you should be able to put it out of your mind. With this being said, it is important to learn the difference between habitual hunger and true hunger as there may be a time when you legitimately need to end your fast early if your body is just not prepared to go the distance.

Fast for the right reasons: There is any number of previously discussed reasons to pursue an intermittent fasting lifestyle that are perfectly valid but using it as an excuse to cover up deeper issues related to a desire to not consume enough calories or to cover up a bingeing and purging cycle are not on the list. Before you make the decision to try intermittent fasting it is important you have a clear idea that you possess the willpower to not just to prevent yourself from eating but to never go an unhealthy amount of time without eating as well.

Conclusion

Thank you for making it through to the end of *Intermittent Fasting for Women: Burn Fat in Less Than 30 Days With Serious Permanent Weight Loss in Very Simple, Healthy and Easy Scientific Way, Eat More Food and Lose More Weight*, let's hope it was informative and able to provide you with all of the tools you need to achieve your goals, whatever it is that they may be. Just because you've finished this book doesn't mean there is nothing left to learn on the topic, expanding your horizons is the only way to find the mastery you seek.

It is important to understand that, when it comes to practicing intermittent fasting in the long-term, no two people are going to respond to the process in the same way. Practically, what this means is that you are going to want to actively strive to do your best to avoid pushing body towards anything remotely resembling a breaking point just because you want to lose as much weight as possible no matter what. After all, intermittent fasting isn't a race and you won't receive a medal for coming in first place. Work up to the level of fasting that you are comfortable with, your body will thank you.

As long as you keep that in mind, however, then it is time to stop reading to and to get ready to get started changing your lifestyle for the better. There are plenty of different types of intermittent fasting out there and as long as you have the dedication and mental fortitude to fast for at least 12 hours then there is nothing you can't do. As long as you settle in for the long haul, and don't expect too much too soon, there is no reason you can't be well on your way to a healthier, happier, life in just one month.

Finally, if you found this book useful in any way, a review is always appreciated!

Description

The practice of intermittent fasting has been around for countless centuries and used for nearly as many different purposes.

However, the reason that most people have heard about the practice these days is thanks to its proven ability to help those who practice it lose weight and keep it off in the long-term while at the same time feeling more energized than they have in years.

The best part?

Getting into the intermittent fasting lifestyle doesn't require you to give up the foods you love or even eat fewer calories per meal!

In fact, the most commonly used type of intermittent fasting makes it possible for those who practice it to skip breakfast before eating two meals later in the day. This type of lifestyle change is ideal for those who find themselves having trouble sticking with a stricter diet plan as it doesn't take much of a change to start seeing serious results, as opposed to being forced to change everything all at once.

If you like what you've heard so far, then *Intermittent Fasting for Women: Burn Fat in Less Than 30 Days with Serious Permanent Weight Loss in Very Simple, Healthy and Easy Scientific Way, Eat More Food and Lose More Weight* is the book you have been waiting for.

Inside you will find:

- Health concerns that women need to keep in mind to practice intermittent fasting successfully.
- Why you should lose no more than 0.5 Kg per week.

- Guides for several types of intermittent fasting specifically tailored to help women find success
- Tips for adding exercise to an intermittent fasting plan without losing yourself to hunger
- Easy ways to make the transition to an intermittent fasting lifestyle as easy as possible
- ***And more...***

www.ingramcontent.com/pod-product-compliance
Lightning Source LLC
Chambersburg PA
CBHW072146020426
42334CB00018B/1904